Does money matter?

Does money matter?

Older people's views of their monetary resources

Glenda Cook, Jan Reed, Susan Childs and Amanda Hall

JR
JOSEPH
ROWNTREE
FOUNDATION

The **Joseph Rowntree Foundation** has supported this project as part of its programme of research and innovative development projects, which it hopes will be of value to policy makers, practitioners and service users. The facts presented and views expressed in this report are, however, those of the authors and not necessarily those of the Foundation.

Joseph Rowntree Foundation
The Homestead
40 Water End
York YO30 6WP
Website: www.jrf.org.uk

First published 2004 by the Joseph Rowntree Foundation

ISBN 1 85935 159 X (paperback)
ISBN 1 85935 160 3 (pdf: available at www.jrf.org.uk)

A CIP catalogue record for this report is available from the British Library.

Cover design by Adkins Design

Prepared and printed by:
York Publishing Services Ltd
64 Hallfield Road
Layerthorpe
York
YO31 7ZQ
Tel: 01904 430033 Fax: 01904 430868 Website: www.yps-publishing.co.uk

Further copies of this report, or any other JRF publication, can be obtained either from the JRF website (www.jrf.org.uk/bookshop/) or from our distributor, York Publishing Services Ltd, at the above address.

CONTENTS

Acknowledgements

This project was funded by the Joseph Rowntree Foundation. The study was carried out by two research centres, CCOP (Centre for Care of Older People) and IMRI (Information Management Research Institute), both based at Northumbria University. CCOP undertakes research that gives a voice to older people and has a commitment to multi-disciplinary research and to developing links with local agencies and organisations in statutory and non-statutory sectors. The research, development and consultancy activity of IMRI focuses on the people-centred aspects of the design, development and evaluation of information systems and services in a wide range of human and organisational contexts. Members of the research team were:

- Glenda Cook (Centre for Care of Older People, Northumbria University)
- Professor Jan Reed (Centre for Care of Older People, Northumbria University)
- Susan Childs (Information Management Research Institute, Northumbria University)
- Amanda Hall (Information Management Research Institute, Northumbria University).

Members of the Expert Panel were:

- Alan Curry (Age Concern, Newcastle)
- Peter Fulton (Older Persons' Champion, South Tees Hospitals NHS Trust)
- Sheila Rooney (Social Policy Coordinator, Washington Citizens Advice Bureau)
- Robert Weiner (Liaison Officer, North East Pre-retirement Association).

Key informants were:

- older people from the following groups:
  1 members of a London-based leisure and educational voluntary group for the over 50s
  2 attendees of a social services day centre
  3 residential home residents
  4 nursing home residents
- Vera Bolter (Better Government for Older People, Newcastle)
- Jayne Curry (Deputy Care at Home Manager, Age Concern, Newcastle)
- Dr Mary Davies (Director, Pre-retirement Association)
- Sue Pearson (Chief Executive, Age Concern, Newcastle)
- Ruth Robson (Secretary of the Ryton Pathfinders)

- Irene Smith (Bureau Manager, Citizens Advice Bureau, Washington)
- Jack White (Treasurer and Membership Secretary, National Pensioners Association, UK)
- Professor John Veit-Wilson (Sociology and Social Policy, University of Newcastle)
- Richard Wilson (Policy Officer on Income, Help the Aged).

Scott Matthews of the Nursing, Midwives and Allied Health Professionals (NMAHP) Research and Development Unit at Northumbria University acted as editorial adviser for the report.

1 Introduction

This project was commissioned by the Joseph Rowntree Foundation to provide a review of the literature concerning the question 'Does money matter to older people?'. Often, it is assumed that money does matter, and the focus of attention rests on how much money people have and what they use their money for. The emphasis on these issues gives rise to a line of enquiry about measuring income and expenditure, and mapping how money is spent. Although such enquiries have generated valuable information about the financial circumstances of older people, they do not address the ways in which older people live their lives in those conditions. In contrast to this, the question posed by the commissioners is qualitatively different as it seeks to explore how older people view their financial circumstances, how they use their money and what needs they feel should be met. These are important issues to explore in a society where financial resources are identified as antecedent to participation and consumer spending power is viewed as a central part of having choice and control. In this society, such values are highly regarded and associated with notions of citizenship.

The expression 'older people' is used throughout this report to refer to those who have reached the chronological age of eligibility for the state pension. Use of this term serves the purpose of creating a framework to identify the population of interest to the study, but it does not reflect the diverse financial circumstances of this group of people. Older people include the poorest people in the country, particularly those over the age of 75, and those who have a high financial status. Any conclusions that are drawn, therefore, have to address this diversity.

The brief privileged the views of older people by focusing on their experiences and their perceptions of the role money had in shaping their lives. In keeping with the spirit of the commissioning process, the design of the literature search was developed with older people and the discussions that we had with them were used to inform every aspect of the study. This report is reflective of this process. Specific topics were identified in the brief: the financial resources needed to participate fully in society, paying for care, and debates about cash or care. The literature review also included those issues that were identified through our conversations with older people. This resulted in a wide-ranging review of literature from different disciplines because the issues that were identified as important to older people did not fall neatly into the traditional ways of categorising literature according to academic disciplines. Their concerns cut across the boundaries of economics, sociology, gerontology, health and psychology. In addition to this, the findings arising from the review of the literature do not merely report on what is known or what has been studied about the role of money in later life as would be the case in an orthodox literature review. The findings include the comments and the ideas that the participants expressed throughout the study to give them a voice of equal importance to the voice of policy makers and researchers that is documented in the literature.

The study had two strands that fed into each other. One strand included processes to capture the ideas that older people have about whether money matters, why it matters and how it matters. Resources and time constraints did not allow us to carry out an extensive exploration of older people's ideas. This activity was therefore restricted to small, easily accessible groups of older people: those who could travel to Northumbria University to take part in a discussion and those who were able to take part in a telephone discussion about issues of concern to the study. The second strand involved procedures to identify, locate and review literature about the topics that were highlighted by the participants.

The activities that were involved in each strand took place concurrently and the knowledge that was acquired as a result informed the next stage of data collection or analysis of the data that had been acquired. Detailed description of these processes is presented in the methodology section (Chapter 2) of the report. Figure 1 gives the reader an overview of how the study was conducted and portrays how the two strands of the study were interrelated.

One of the fundamental questions that was considered throughout this study was 'If money matters to the way that people live, are older people different?'. It was concluded that older people do have different concerns. Younger people are living through a stage of their life that is concerned with asset accumulation. They have the potential to increase their income and spend a large proportion of their income on those things that are associated with young and middle adulthood such as mortgages, or bringing up children. By contrast, older people have entered a period of their life when the potential to increase their income is minimal. They experience asset dispersal and their spending priorities are concerned with resourcing something meaningful to do in their later years, and financing aids, equipment, household adaptations and paying for care. This report aims to recognise and understand how older people use their money and what needs they feel should be met. By doing this, the report will contribute to a knowledge base that is important to enable the development of research, policies and practices that are grounded in the expectations and concerns of older people.

Figure 1 The two strands of the study

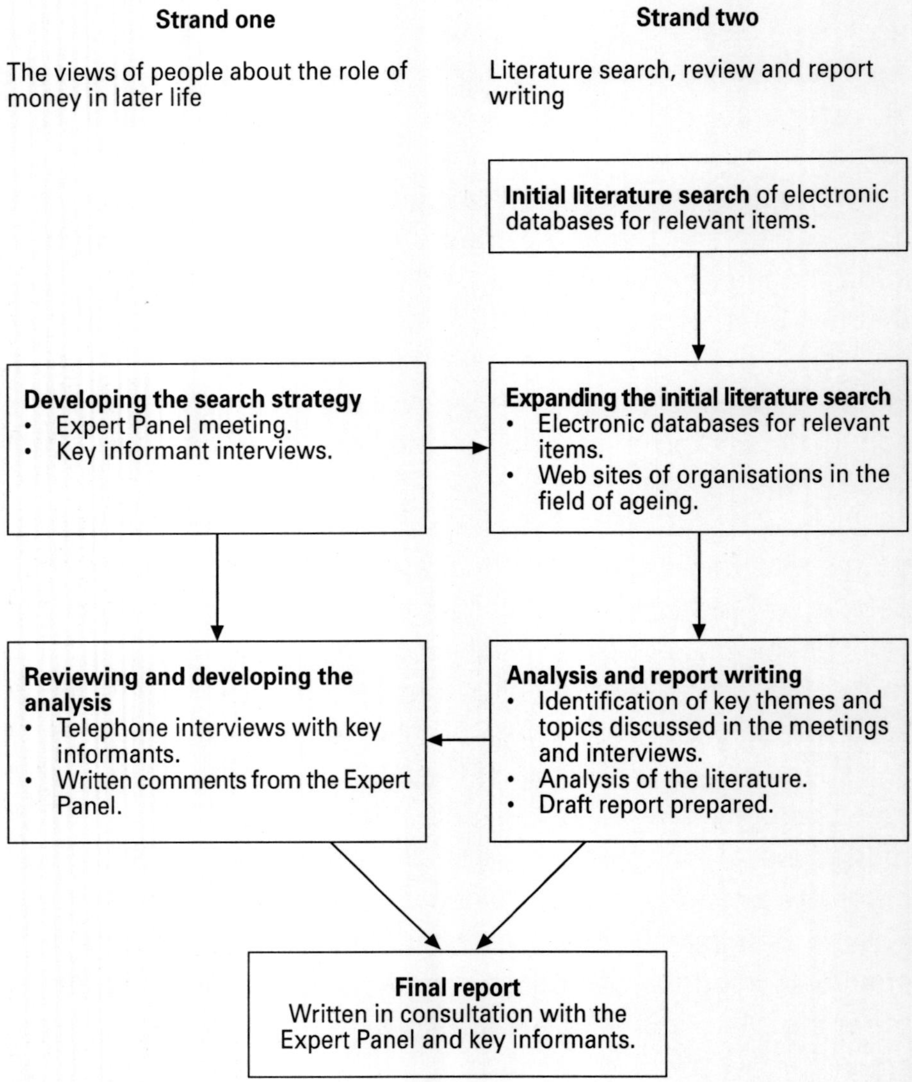

2 METHODOLOGY

The study was designed to ground the literature review in the experiences of older people, and those working with them, to develop an understanding of the ways in which older people need and desire financial support. To do this, the process of retrieving and reviewing the literature was iterative. We would conduct a search, feedback the results, then extend or amend the search in the light of people's comments. This provided opportunities to go back to the initial stage of searching the literature when new topics and issues were introduced by those taking part in the study. This approach stands in contrast with the traditional, sequential process of searching the electronic databases, sifting the outcomes of the search, retrieving relevant literature, analysing it and reporting on the findings. The process will be described to give the reader a detailed account of how the literature was identified and subsequently reviewed.

Strand one: eliciting the views of older people about the role of money in later life

As shown in Figure 1 in Chapter 1, this strand of the study involved discussions and interviews with older people, and with those working with them, to help us to identify key topics concerning the role of money in later life and to search for relevant literature. We were able to do this by organising an Expert Panel meeting with those who were known to the research team and who could travel to take part. We were also able to conduct group and individual interviews with older people who acted as key informants to the study. Analysis of the Expert Panel and key informant discussions resulted in identification of a number of themes that reflected the key issues for older people with respect to money.

These themes were used as a framework for the review of the literature that was identified. The Expert Panel and key informants were able to give us comments on our review of the literature and to participate in the writing of this report. The following sections describe the conversations that we had with these participants and the processes that we used to analyse this information.

The Expert Panel meeting

Members of the Expert Panel are listed in the Acknowledgements at the front of this report. The Panel was created to identify key issues and concerns relating to the role of money in later life. When they met the following topics were discussed.

- What is a basic income?
- How do older people use their money?
- What needs should be met?
- What strategies do older people employ to manage their financial circumstances?
- What sources of financial support have been generated for later life and what financial sources do older people have access to?

- Paying for personal, social and health care and adaptations to the home.
- What role does money play in promoting independence and autonomy in later life?
- What funding do older people desire to enable them to address their personal and health care needs?

This section of the meeting lasted for three-and-half hours, and the entire discussion was tape-recorded and transcribed verbatim in preparation for analysis.

Following exploration of the above topics, the Panel was asked to identify search words and phrases that would refine and expand the initial list that had been developed by the research team. These words are important because the process of locating literature is done largely by searching databases using specific search terms and keywords. The following terms were identified:

- basic income
- basic needs
- budget management
- budget standards
- finance plus advocacy
- financial autonomy
- financial gerontology
- financial literacy

- financial strategies
- financial well-being
- income plus autonomy
- minimal income
- personal budgets
- poverty plus review/overview
- social care plus money/finances
- social exclusion plus money/finances
- spending patterns.

The Panel was also asked to identify key authors who had been influential in shaping their thinking about the role of money in later life. The following authors were identified and the names were used to conduct a search of the databases for literature that had been written by them:

- Jonathon Bradshaw
- Geoff Femister
- Mary Gilhooly (Paisley)
- Michael Hill
- Peter Townsend

- John Veit-Wilson
- Michael Younge.

The discussion moved on to explore ways to identify and access grey literature (see section headed 'Sources and types of material' later in this chapter for discussion of this type of literature). In addition to the Panel members contributing literature that they had acquired (such as conference abstracts and articles, and organisational reports), suggestions were made to search web sites and approach organisations to retrieve relevant literature. Identified organisations were:

- Age Concern
- Child Poverty Action Group
- Church Poverty Action Group
- Citizens Advice Bureau
- Department of Social Security
- Edinburgh Waverly papers
- General Household Survey
- Help the Aged
- Joseph Rowntree Foundation
- Magistrates' Association
- National Association of Citizens Advice Bureaux (NACAB)

- National Pensioners Association
- National Pensioners Convention
- NIACE (National Institute for Adult Continuing Education)
- Pre-retirement Association
- Social Trends.

At the end of the meeting, Panel members agreed to comment on our analysis of this discussion and review of the literature.

Key informants' interviews

Older people were invited to take part in a group or individual interview to discuss their personal experiences of growing old in the UK and the role that money had played in shaping their experiences. Twenty-two older people participated in the following interviews.

- Two group interviews were carried out with older people who were members of a leisure and educational voluntary group for those over 50 in London (n = 10).
- One group interview was held with six older people living in a residential care home in Newcastle-upon-Tyne.
- One group interview was held with four older people who attended a social services day centre in Newcastle-upon-Tyne.
- Two individual interviews were carried out with nursing home residents, as they were unable to take part in group interviews.

These interviews were tape-recorded and transcribed verbatim in preparation for analysis.

Analysis of the Expert Panel meeting and interview data

The transcripts were read and standard methods of open coding were used to identify the topics, issues and themes that were discussed by the participants. At this stage of the project, the findings from the data analysis included a high proportion of direct extracts from the interviews in an attempt to accurately portray the views of the participants. This also created a way for the project team to return to the original data to check out new understandings that had been acquired during reading of the literature.

Consultation and development of the final report

As the project team carried out the process of analysing the transcripts and reviewing the literature, the possibility that the voice of the academic may overshadow the voice of others who were involved in the development of the final report was a real concern. To address this, the report was drafted and distributed to members of the Expert Panel for consultation. While the project team waited for their feedback, telephone and face-to-face interviews (n = 9) were carried out with representatives of the organisations identified by the Expert Panel and authors who had been highlighted during the literature search (see the list of key informants in the Acknowledgements at the front of this report). During the interviews, the interviewees' views about the findings were explored.

Strand two: searching for and reviewing the literature

The second strand of the study involved searching and selecting the literature, which was informed by the conversations and discussions that we had with older people, and by previous reading and work in the area. This stage had two elements to it: first, the retrieval of material from electronic databases, to form a list of papers and items, and then a second process where these lists were scrutinised and relevant items were selected for acquisition (copies were obtained through inter-library loans or electronic journals). Uncovering relevant material through searching literature is not a straightforward activity. Between authors writing material and its inclusion in a database there is a complex process whereby, at each stage, decisions are made about what an item is about.

Sources and types of material

There are issues about what is published and how it is made available to potential readers. Academic and professional literature is usually published in an organised way through journals, books, reports of conferences, etc. These items are managed by commercial publishers who ensure that potential readers can gain access to the literature. They achieve this by labelling each item with full bibliographic information, making it available for purchase, distribution and promotion to database producers.

Databases are commercially developed for specific audiences or markets. They are often specialised, including only material from a limited number of journals that have established records containing relevant material of a suitable quality. When an item is included in a database, keywords or search terms are assigned. This means that it can be searched under author, title, date, or subject heading (keywords), depending on the database and its structure.

All these processes take time. It can take many months, or even years, before a written article is actually published in a journal. It can then take a similar period of time before an article appears in a database, if it ever does. Hence, databases will not necessarily contain the most up-to-date material.

There is another type of literature, grey literature, which is usually not attainable through conventional publication and retrieval systems. However, such literature can often contain very useful information, particularly about projects and services provided by individual organisations and research projects, or in specific localities. It consists of locally produced reports, meeting papers, discussion and policy documents, etc.

Grey literature can be variable in the bibliographic details that are given. While some items are described fully, others might lack an author's name, even a date, and it can be unclear who the publisher is (i.e. which organisation has produced it). Grey literature is not recorded in databases. Nor is it peer-reviewed. Usually, the author and producer do not take even the simple step of depositing their work with the British Library so that it will appear in the national British Library catalogue and be available through inter-library loan. The normal method of 'publication' of grey literature is the in-house production of a small number of copies that are sent to a restricted list of people. The content of the literature could be confidential or organisationally sensitive, which will restrict the initial audience even further. A wider or future audience is not catered for.

Search strategy in this study

In searching and locating items, one has to negotiate all the complexities discussed above. This involves understanding the limitations of databases, the way in which they use search terms and the material they index. It also involves understanding the environment in which research and development takes place, in so far as research gets funding only if it fits in with funders' priorities and goals, and their model of the world. Medical research funders would therefore fund research that accords with their priorities and uses terms that fit with their language. In this respect, they operate in the same way as social scientific research funders. As older people are not usually funders of research, and are only just beginning to have a say in research priorities, it is not surprising that the search terms and keywords in databases may not fit their models of knowledge.

The process of identifying and selecting items to fit the project brief therefore involves processes of translation and interpretation backed up by an understanding of the way in which information becomes available, and ways in which it can be accessed. The terms of the project brief had to be interpreted in the light of database search terms and author keywords. This process relied on the knowledge that the research team had of literature searching and of the topic being explored. From this, it was possible to make judgements about the relevance of material and also to generate items for inclusion in the review based on the researcher's expertise in this area.

The subject of the brief 'Does money matter?' uses concepts that are difficult to describe precisely and additionally uses words and phrases that have general, wide-ranging usage. If you are looking for keywords to describe older people, there are many available, including older/old, ageing/aged, elderly, retired, senior (linked with people/person/citizen), geriatrics, pensioners. The availability of keywords for financial topics is much wider, including income, finances/financial, benefits, pensions, costs, expenditure, spending, poverty/poorer, wealth, better-off, as a few examples. These words then have to be combined together in a meaningful way to create a final, full-search strategy. Often, when searching using terms like these, items are found that are wholly irrelevant to the project topic. This is because these common words are of course used to mean different things in different contexts. For example, a search for 'aged' and 'healthy' as key words may find items about 'aged expectant mothers' (who are pregnant but older than in their early 20s) and a 'healthy pregnancy'. Such irrelevant items are often called 'false hits'.

In searching, there is always a balance between getting relevant items and avoiding irrelevant items. If you aim for a precise, specific search you will retrieve less irrelevant items, but with the downside that you will have excluded relevant items in the process. If you go for a sensitive search, to try to retrieve as many relevant items as possible, then the downside is that you will also retrieve many irrelevant items. One point to remember is that, for the many reasons discussed above, even the most sensitive search will never find all the relevant items that exist in the database being searched.

A different search process was needed for grey literature as databases, on the whole, cannot be used. Traditional (non-electronic) methods are appropriate here. These include looking in the reference lists of articles and books to see what information sources the authors used (which could include grey literature as well as academic literature), and asking experts in the topic for their recommendations of grey literature. These traditional methods can be powerful approaches and can find very useful information, but they are clearly only scratching at the surface of the grey literature that must exist. Traditional methods are also useful in searching for academic literature to fill some of the gaps in coverage that we have discussed and will always occur in a literature search. They form part of the procedures for undertaking a systematic review too (see later definition).

Our approach was to go for a more sensitive search and accept that we would retrieve a number of irrelevant items too. The results of a pilot search are given in the Appendix, which shows how large a number of items were initially retrieved. We dealt with these by a step-wise selection process whereby two members of the project team looked at the results independently, then compared their choice and came to an agreement through discussion. For the first stage, the obvious 'false hits' were discarded. In the second stage, less obvious irrelevant items were discarded, for example those that, on more detailed reading, were irrelevant, or those that, though broadly in the topic area, did not meet the specific requirements of the project brief.

A final point will set the literature review for this project in context with other literature reviews. In the health field, there is a growing use of systematic reviews of the literature. These use detailed procedures that aim for a more comprehensive and objective search and selection of the literature (NHS CRD, 2001). However, systematic reviews are very costly in terms of money and staff time. They can cost tens of thousands of pounds and can take up to a year or more to complete, with a person being involved full-time, and with other staff on a part-time basis.

The literature search that was carried out focused on accessing both published material and grey literature that related to the topics and issues that were identified by the Expert Panel and the key informants. As we were restricted by the timescale that we were set to complete this study, we commenced an initial search of the literature using search terms and keywords that were included in the brief that had been prepared by the commissioners of the study. The initial search was expanded following the Expert Panel meeting and key informant interviews. Details of the process of literature searching are shown in Box 1.

The initial searches were carried out on the following databases:

- AMED (Allied and Complementary Medicine)
- CINAHL (Nursing and Allied Health)

Box 1 Literature searching and selection

Identifying literature

- Initial literature search: project team brainstorm of search terms and initial search from selected databases conducted.
- Expanding the initial search following the Expert Panel meeting and key informant interviews: secondary search of databases using additional databases and expanded search terms/keywords.
- Web sites of key organisations in the field of ageing were checked for relevant material.

Selecting the literature

- Duplicate references and false hits removed.
- Selection of literature that reflected the themes that were identified from analysis of the meetings and interviews.

- EBM Reviews – Cochrane Controlled Trials Register
- Cochrane Reviews.

(Note: Medline was not used as the large number of hits retrieved made searching within the project constraints unfeasible and as the focus of this database was not judged to be directly relevant to the research question.)

The search strategy retrieved any English language articles that contained terms (one or more) from each of the lists below. The lists were designed to capture the concepts of 'older people' and 'money' respectively:

- older people, elderly people, geriatric(s), retired, retirement, senior citizen(s), pensioner(s)
- money, income(s), expenditure, spending, financial, finances, payment(s), benefits, purchasing).

Following removal of duplicates, 585 references were retrieved during the initial search of the databases. A large proportion of false hits were obtained during the initial search and these had to be discarded by hand. For example, articles about the impact of low income on the lives of young children were identified. Discarding false hits and selecting relevant items was achieved by two members of the project team independently reviewing the full computer record (bibliographic details, abstract and keywords) of each item. They then discussed their selections and reached a consensus. The final selection comprised 36 items. Full-text versions of these articles were obtained and read.

Expanding the initial literature search

Following analysis of the Expert Panel meeting and key informant interviews, it was identified that the references obtained during the initial search of the literature were missing the social science dimension. It was decided that a search on a database such as the Social Sciences Citation Index was required to address the gap in the literature that had been identified. A subject search was carried out on the Social Sciences Citation Index (SSCI) and the other databases included in the initial search using the identified search terms from the conversations that we had with the Expert Panel and key informants. Three-hundred-and-six references were retrieved. Using the same process of independent selection as described above, six items were selected for inclusion in the literature review.

Author and citation searches (i.e. searches that identified papers that cited these authors) were carried out on the key authors identified during the Expert Panel meeting and 29 references were retrieved. Using the process of independent selection, 11 items were selected.

These two sets of selected references were combined and full-text version of these articles were obtained and read.

The web sites of key organisations in the field of ageing were checked for relevant literature. Policy documents, policy position papers, responses to government calls for consultation, etc. were identified and appropriate ones selected for review. However, in some cases, older documents were not available on the web sites. Additionally, there were information leaflets/books geared to the older person themselves. These were not selected for review.

Members of the Expert Panel identified items of grey literature that were read and then selected for inclusion in the review.

Literature review

All of the literature that had been retrieved was read and annotated in preparation for the analysis that followed. This commenced with categorising the literature according to the codes that had been developed from analysis of the interview and meeting data. The assignment of categories was complex. Some of the literature addressed a specific category that had been developed, whereas other pieces cut across more than one category. In the latter situation, more than one category was assigned to a particular article. The complexity of this process was increased because the language used by the participants did not necessarily correspond with the language found in the literature. Consequently, the codes were extended to bridge the gaps between academic and lay language where this existed.

Following this, all the literature within a category was re-read and the content was used to extend or refine the findings that had been derived from analysis of the interview and meeting data. The results of this process are reported in the following sections of the report.

3 Findings

The importance of money in later life

Undoubtedly, the answer to the question 'Does money matter?' is yes of course it matters – income has a major influence on standard of living and well-being in later life. An older person's perception of the quality of their life is influenced by many factors including health and functional status, meaningful activity, relationships and social support, as well as financial situation (Prestoy, 1993; Gnich and Gilhooly, 1997; Ozawa and Lum, 1997; Walters and Charles, 1997; Bryant *et al.*, 2001). For older people, financial security that enhances the quality of their life refers to 'having enough to do what they want to do when they want to do it' (Prestoy, 1993, p. 166). In other words, financial security means having enough money to meet daily needs, while allowing for entertainment and leisure activities, in contrast to living below, on, or just above the poverty level.

Determining what is or is not 'enough' is inherently value laden because what is adequate to one person may be totally inadequate to another. Yet, there needs to be some way of measuring adequacy as this knowledge is crucial to decisions about income needs following retirement. Recent studies commissioned by Age Concern and the Family Budget Unit have attempted to do this by quantifying how much income an older person requires to avoid living in poverty (this is called 'the Low Cost but Acceptable Standard'). The authors suggest that this equates to the poverty threshold and generally people aim higher than this

(Parker, 2000). Hence, their following study focused on estimating the income required to reach a reasonable standard of living ('the Modest but Adequate Standard', Age Concern, 2002b). This standard allows for a healthy diet, durables that 50 per cent of similar households would possess and an inexpensive holiday. The authors argue that this budget provides the opportunity to participate fully in society (Parker, 2002). The Expert Panel welcomed these recent attempts to translate the concept of a basic income into living costs, as this enabled individuals living in different circumstances to make judgements about their financial status according to some objective rather than subjective measure. They argued that perceptions of a basic income did vary and this was influenced by previous experience. As one participant said:

> To me the basic income would vary from person to person depending on what they had been used to throughout their life before retirement.

> Basic spending varies from person to person in accordance with the lifestyle they have enjoyed before they retired and the size of their income. This changes following retirement and adaptations have to be made according to the amount of money available to spend.

These ideas suggest that notions of a basic income are associated with maintaining the financial status acquired throughout life. For some, living on a meagre income reflects their life's experiences whereas others may have enjoyed continuous employment resulting in a steady income. The majority of people experience a decline in their income after retirement (Disney *et al.*, 1978; Bardasi and Jenkins, 2002). Nonetheless, maintaining the financial status that they have experienced throughout life is an important factor with respect to experiencing well-being after retirement (George, 1992; Mein *et al.*, 1998, 2000). Income security, the degree to which a person's customary standard of living is protected from the ups and downs of economic circumstance, has a major influence on financial status (Atchley, 1997). The literature is rich with debates about the relative value of retirement income and how decreases in this have a negative impact on the lives of older people (see, for example, Ozawa and Lum, 1998; Bradshaw, 2000; Parker, 2000; Marmot and Wilkinson, 2001; Whetstone, 2002). Johnson *et al.* (1998), in their analysis of the Retirement Survey data collected in 1988/89 and 1994, found that there is a strong relationship between pension level and the probability of indexation. That is, pensions that start low are less likely than higher pensions to keep up with inflation. Consequently, the real value of low incomes decreases over time as a result of poor indexation.

Analysis of recent trends suggests that the older population is becoming increasingly dichotomised into rich and poor, with the oldest pensioners tending to be poorer than those more recently retired (Gnich and Gilhooly, 1997; Villa *et al.*, 1997; Johnson *et al.*, 1998). Although social security wealth is almost universal, other assets such as financial and housing wealth, and the value of occupational and personal pensions are much more unevenly distributed (Disney *et al.*, 1998). In the UK, it is argued that low incomes are expected and accepted as being part of old age (Evans and Falkingham, 1997; Mein *et al.*, 2000). This is supported by the statistics collated by the Department of Works and Pensions (2001), which indicate that a quarter of all pensioners, approximately 2.75 million, occupy the bottom quintile of income distribution. Though this is the case, income growth among individuals of pensionable age is occurring more than for the population as a whole. Since the damage done by poverty has been widely acknowledged, the plight of older people is a matter for concern since they are disproportionately represented in the lower income bracket. There is also much evidence that the very old, women, immigrants and those with broken work records or a long history of low-paid work are over-represented in this group (Bartlett, 2001; Bardasi and Jenkins, 2002). Recent debates, however, have shifted attention from this to the effect of inequality on health. For example, Marmot and Wilkinson (2001) point to the findings from the Whitehall studies on British civil servants, which indicate that:

> ... there is a gradient in health among those who are not poor, indicating that the higher the socio-economic position, the lower the morbidity and mortality ... there is a strong relation between mortality and income inequalities.
>
> (Marmot and Wilkinson, 2001, p. 1233)

The combination of low income and increasing income inequality, therefore, has resulted in exposures that have a significant negative impact on the health and well-being of older people.

Financial literacy

Entering retirement is a significant time when concerns about managing on a reduced income or spending the capital acquired throughout life arise. Every source of income – state/occupational/private pension, state benefits, investments and savings – has complex rules and processes to negotiate (Hedges, 1998).

Consequently, new skills and knowledge are needed to enable the person to make informed judgements and to take effective decisions about the use and management of their money. The complex income structures of older people require highly developed analytical and numeracy skills to enable them to understand what their regular income is and how this may change, how to access their capital and how to estimate financial needs in the future (NIACE, 2001). The bewildering range of financial choices, poor quality information, poor advice, changes to taxation rules, hybridisation of financial services and the development of e-commerce compounds the difficulty in understanding financial resources (Lord, 2001).

Box 2 People do not always know what they are entitled to and do not claim their money – an example given by a member of the Expert Panel

> The pension department in the place I worked in write out every year in April to say that the cost of living has gone up so much, so you are going to get that much more money. They got back a letter from a widow saying 'well that's not really good for me' and could she please have the money. She did not want this rise – could she please have the money. The pensions department looked into this to see what was going on. In fact her husband had died two years previously. There was something like £10,000 in his bank account and that was actually hers, from her widow's pension. She didn't think that she was entitled to it ... she had been living off the state pension for the last few years. They had to explain to her that that was a widow's pension and it was hers.

In the literature, there is evidence that people, generally, are not financially literate to competently manage their monetary resources (Cutler, 1997; Financial Services Authority, 1998; Department for Education and Employment, 1999; Walker and

Davies, 2001). Older people have been found to experience some or extreme difficulty in understanding their finances, including banking, credit cards and bills (NIACE, 2002). They are particularly challenged by the necessity to make well-informed decisions about their relatively fixed income, and sometimes this takes place when physical and mental abilities are declining, which affects their ability to make sound judgements. A generalised concern has also arisen about older women who experience termination of their relationship or are widowed. They may have been responsible for making short-term financial decisions throughout their marriage, however the responsibility for longer-term decisions may have rested with their partner. They therefore face a steep learning curve in their new circumstances (Bartlett, 2001).

Such generalisations do highlight important issues about the way in which older people understand and manage their money. Older people, however, are a diverse group whose skills are equally varied. This was given little attention in the literature that we identified and the participants were keen to reflect the range of abilities of older people:

> Most of my acquaintances, who are in their 60s and 70s are quite capable of handling their finances as they are used to having their salaries paid directly into bank accounts.

According to NIACE (2001, 2002), older people tend to rely on those who support them to obtain information and advise their financial decisions as there is a general mistrust of financial suppliers and their advisers. As the problems of financial literacy pervade the entire population, this may not lead to the best financial decisions for the older person. They need support to make sense of all the financial information that they confront and, in recent years, many initiatives have been developed with the aim of increasing financial competency of older people. Examples of these initiatives include the 'Financial literacy and older people project' (FLOP) and 'It doesn't add up' project, undertaken by NIACE. These contributed towards a deeper understanding of the issues faced by older people and towards the development of teaching materials for financial learning programmes tailored to their needs. Many schemes have been created to target people who are making major financial decisions as they face the transition to retirement. The North East Pre-retirement workshops are an example of this, which include input from independent financial advisers, the Pensions Service and Inland Revenue. Many advice agencies across the country are now targeting older people to provide advice on welfare benefits. For example, the Washington Citizens Advice Bureau has recently appointed specialist debt and benefit workers who have a detailed understanding of the financial issues faced by older people in recognition of their need for support with these problems.

These developments have focused on the information needs of older people and increasing support to help older people to make sense of it in the context of their own circumstances. In addition to what has been developed, the Expert Panel suggested that independent financial advocacy and advisory services were needed to support older people to independently manage their own finances.

While initiatives have been developed to address the needs of older people, attention has also been given to develop ways to enable people to become financially literate at a younger age. A few examples can be given. Notably, financial education has been introduced to the National Curriculum. Personnel departments in many organisations have extended their role to give money education and advice. The Pre-retirement Association (2000) has published 'best practice' guidelines for employers on the subject of financial education. (These were designed to enable employees to engage in pension planning in the context of financial and lifestyle planning.) Meanwhile, there are calls for all financial information to be 'financially literacy proofed' (Lord, 2001). The key objective of these initiatives is to raise general awareness of the need for financial literacy and to develop the relevant competencies to manage money. This may result in a situation whereby those entering retirement are better prepared to face the challenges of financial decisions in later life.

Harsh times: living on a low income

Members of the Expert Panel and the key informants stressed that having an adequate income was important. Older people would otherwise experience constant worry and anxiety about how they would be able to meet the financial demands of maintaining adequate diet, clothing, housing and heating. Unlike other groups in society, older people have limited opportunity to alter their financial position, as they have minimal earning power and their ability to earn decreases as age advances. This leads to a situation where they exist on the money that has been acquired throughout life or on state pensions and benefits. Those who have experienced broken work records, a work history of low-paid employment, reduced earning years (as they brought up a family or provided long-term care for others) are particularly disadvantaged. They enter retirement with the prospect of living the following 20 to 30 years on a low income (Villa *et al.*, 1997; Ozawa and Lum, 1998; Walker *et al.*, 2000; Bartlett, 2001; Whetstone, 2002).

The key informants who were reliant on the state retirement pension and benefits, with little or no access to personal savings, described how they managed on what they perceived to be less than a basic income. They experienced a harsh existence. They had to make decisions about buying fresh, nutritious food or 'out-of-date and poor quality food', which enabled them to take part in inexpensive activities or put a little money aside for repairs to their home that may arise in the future. Others spoke of not being able to budget for new clothing and having to request clothing as gifts or to shop at second-hand shops if the need arose.

Modern society has arranged itself in such a way that there is great reliance on transport to access super/hypermarkets that are often located on the periphery of urban districts. While these stores offer a wider range of cheaper, good quality food, the consumer needs to calculate the cost of travel to decide if the savings on the shopping bill merit the additional costs. The ways in which special offers are made available to customers in these stores are often based on multiple buys – the 'buy one get one free' or 'three for the price of two' offers – which are not economical to pensioners who mainly live in smaller households.

Some of the participants lived in housing estates that were far removed from supermarkets. As they were unable to travel to the nearest supermarket because of poor health, limited mobility or the lack of money to fund travel, they purchased their household items and groceries from the local store in their neighbourhood. These items were often more expensive than similar items in the larger stores. Consequently, they faced decisions about purchasing the poorer quality products to reduce the cost knowing that this may have a detrimental effect on their health or cutting back on other day-to-day expenditure such as heating to buy the better food. Many of the participants who were living on a low income described their life as 'living on the breadline'. They were not able to afford 'a little bit of entertainment' or take part in activities that would be fulfilling.

Alongside discussion of their day-to-day experiences of living on low incomes, the key informants spoke of their spending priorities. This involved decisions about spending money on their immediate needs or setting money aside 'for a rainy day' or 'for the next catastrophe'. As they had limited financial resources, the only way to respond to possible crisis situations was to carefully plan for the possibility that one may occur:

> It's not just about the basics, it is about the unexpected disasters ... If the central heating boiler goes or the cooker goes or something like that. It is about having the back-up resources to get them repaired or get them replaced. So it's not just simply weekly expense.

It was difficult, however, to determine when the rainy day had occurred and to decide to spend capital that could not be replaced. Other unpredictable, worse situations may arise in the future and they were concerned about keeping money to enable them to cope with the unknown situation (see Kempson *et al.*, 2002).

Similar circumstances were described by Whetstone (2002) when reporting on an ethnographic study of the lives of 50 people, aged 70 and over, who were living in a deprived area of central London. She noted that the key money-management strategy that the participants in the study adopted was to cut back on non-essential items such as clothing or economising in other ways. Such strategies diminished the social life of older people and contributed to other problems such as poor physical and mental health, loneliness and isolation. Other illustrations of the deprivation that older people who live on a low income experience are found in a range of literature. For example, Palmer *et al.* (2002), when assembling the indicators of income poverty, identified that those who were dependent on a state pension as their main source of income spent a quarter less on food than other pensioners. The fuel picture (Monroe and Marks, 2002) depicts older people as one of the groups in society who experience fuel poverty because of a combination of poor energy efficiency, fuel costs and household income. In addition, Humphrey and Calder (1990) have found that being able to have a telephone was a luxury that many older people could not afford. For many people living in the UK, having a phone in a house is an essential commodity, as it enables easy and quick communication with others (Gordon *et al.*, 2000). For older people, access to a telephone also offers the security that they can maintain contact with others or contact the emergency services when the need arises. In Humphrey and Calder's (1990) study, other unaffordable items included clothes, redecorating and repairing the house, replacing worn out or broken furniture and renewing bedding. This evidence suggests that older people who live on low incomes experience relative deprivation and social exclusion, as they are unable to purchase socially perceived necessities (Howarth *et al.*, 2001). Whetstone (2002, p. 17) concluded that inclusion in wider society requires an 'individual to have access to the range of resources that a majority of their fellow citizens have'.

In addition to living with the reality of social exclusion, this group of older people also experience the effects of doing without and restriction in their day-to-day life. Financia insecurity, diminished control over circumstances, financial dependency, constant stress and anxiety, lower life satisfaction and diminished feelings of self-worth are common experiences (George, 1993; Krause, 1997; Beresford *et al.*, 1999; Ferraro and Su, 1999; Gnich and Gilhooly, 2001). It can be concluded from this that the impact of living on a low income in later life has wide-ranging and serious effects on the quality of an older person's life.

Reducing income further – poor benefit take-up

The previous discussion suggests that many older people are living in financial circumstances where they are eligible for a range of benefits. Yet, there is considerable evidence that benefit eligibility in the elderly population exceeds actual take-up (Corden, 1995; Flately, 1999; Bramley *et al.*, 2000; Parker, 2002).

The implications of this for older people who are living on lower incomes than necessary have focused researchers' and policy makers' attention on understanding the barriers to benefit take-up. These can be broadly categorised as personal and process barriers. Personal barriers include the stigma associated with claiming many benefits and negative images of claimants as 'spongers' or 'scroungers'; the threat that benefit claims present to personal pride and independence; lack of information about eligibility; and a dislike of the procedures that benefit claiming involves. The process barriers include limited information; complex benefit claim processes; problems associated with physical access to and from the benefit claim office; faceless information services; and perceived lack of privacy in benefit agency offices (Costigan *et al.*, 1999; Bramley *et al.*, 2000; Kempson *et al.*, 2002). Although personal and process barriers have been identified, there is little recognition of the physical barriers to benefit take-up. Those with hearing and visual impairments, or those who are unable to complete forms as a consequence of poor literacy skills, have real difficulties in negotiating the processes for claiming. Such barriers require further investigation to understand the problems and to identify ways of overcoming them.

The Expert Panel and key informants referred to similar issues:

> *[Many elderly women]* do not believe that they have the right to anything other than a very basic income. And they will often not even apply for benefits that they are entitled to because they consider them as not applicable to them because they haven't worked you know ... They have to be persuaded that this is something that is applicable to them.

> This is one of my hobby horses. I know elderly ladies who were living on a basic state pension and were unaware that they could claim housing benefit. Consequently, they were starving themselves. There are a lot of problems with benefit claiming, it is a minefield ready to catch the unwary. The battery of forms that have to be filled in to gain entry to the system is intimidating. These forms have to be filled in every year! Surely the Government can devise a simpler procedure.

They suggested that claiming benefits involves learning about what to apply for, who to approach, and what to disclose to gain the greatest eligibility. It also involves learning about 'gateway benefits' that give access to a whole range of other benefits:

> A man, in his 70s ... had existed on the basic state pension since he retired and ... he was entitled to add-on benefits and went through the whole process ... of filling in these forms and got the grand sum of I think about £5.60. He never claimed this because he said, 'I would not stoop to this, it is an insult this amount of money'. We could not persuade him that this was a gateway benefit that enabled him to collect other benefits. The fact that he had gone through this whole degrading process to get such a small amount of money was so humiliating to him that he didn't want to know anything else. He just didn't want to know. We just couldn't persuade him that he had any other rights at all.

These are illustrative examples of the difficulties and the humiliating situations the Expert Panel and the key informants faced during the transition from living an independent, private life to one that involved disclosing personal details to unknown others and being subjected to means testing. They also spoke of the fears they had experienced when applying for benefits with respect to losing the precious little income that they already had. They did not, therefore, apply for other benefits for which they may have been eligible.

There was strength of feeling expressed during the Expert Panel meeting that older people should not be exposed to these humiliating situations: they were, after all, applying for the financial support that they were entitled to. The move to developing personal approaches such as those piloted by the Benefits Agency Better Government for Older People programme were viewed as supportive and having the potential to encourage older people to take up benefits rather than continuing to live in poverty. These initiatives were aimed at improving take-up of benefits and included alerting older people to their eligibility for benefits, establishing information surgeries situated in convenient locations such as high streets, and creating home visiting and dedicated telephone helpline services (Chang *et al.*, 2001; Kempson *et al.*, 2002).

The changes to the payment of benefits via automatic credit transfer that have taken place during 2003 will present new challenges and perhaps new barriers to the take-up of benefits. Older people are concerned that these changes have been introduced with no consultation. The changes to the payment of benefits and pensions have been introduced to give people a wider choice over where to access their benefit cash as part of the Government's social and financial inclusion agenda. From an organisational perspective, this is a cost-effective way of managing the system of benefit payments as administration costs will be reduced. For some older people, these changes will have social and health implications. To those who live alone, going to the post office is a weekly social event and an opportunity to be with other people. When they no longer do this they may become further isolated, lonely and depressed. There will be a cost implication for the individual, as people tend to live nearer to a post office than to a bank. By contrast, those with high levels of disability who experience difficulty in accessing post offices and who rely on someone else to collect their pension and benefits may be helped with the pending changes (Kempson and Whyley, 2001).

The changes will create the need to develop new skills to manage bank accounts and use modern banking technologies (Rooney, 2002). Some older people who have bypassed the computer society will be directly launched into it and they will be challenged to develop computer skills. In response to these difficulties, telephone support lines and guidance documents are available to support people with the new payment systems. Help the Aged is concerned that older people require additional support to cope with these changes and they are developing an information leaflet that provides advice and guidance specifically aimed at this population.

To address the attitudinal barriers to the take-up of benefits, Costigan *et al.* (1999) have suggested that making income support an automatic payment, and having a single claim for all benefits, would reduce the complexity of the current system. Although these strategies have not been widely debated, they are worthy of attention because the approaches discussed above have focused primarily on access, information and payment issues. People's perceptions of claiming benefits are highly negative and this is the major barrier to benefit take-up that contributes to older people living on incomes that are lower than necessary.

The poverty trap

According to Villa *et al.* (1997), financial security arises from a combination of savings, a pension and social security. During their working years, many people attempt to accumulate assets and contribute to pension schemes in the belief that they are working towards financial security for their later years. However, those at the lower end of the salary scales generate moderate investments and perhaps a small pension that is enough to bring their income above the point that they would qualify for income support and means-tested benefits. In comparison to those qualifying for minimum income guarantee, they are little better off than those reliant on means-tested benefits, if not in a worse financial situation – worse, that is, as a consequence of their lifetime effort to set aside money for the purposes of being able to experience an anxiety-free and comfortable old age (Hedges, 1998; Parker, 2002; Whetstone, 2002).

This situation has come to be known as the poverty trap – a situation that does not reward work and savings. As Bradshaw (2000) argues, it may be difficult to convince the most affected groups in society to continue contributing to a private pension scheme in this situation. In response, the Government has implemented initiatives, such as changes to the capital rules that were introduced in April 2001 and the Pension Credit that was introduced in October 2003. Though Age Concern welcomes these initiatives, it argues that fundamental changes to the basic pension are required to ensure that it covers basic living costs and that it is upgraded annually in line with general living standards (Parker, 2000; Age Concern, 2001a, 2001b). Evandrou and Falkingham (1993) have argued that the changes that were made to the annual process of pension adjustments, which were introduced in 1980, subsequently led to a decrease in the relative value of the state pension. Their calculations led them to conclude that, if the system remained unchanged, the state pension would be worth only 10 per cent of average earnings by 2020.

For some affected by the poverty trap, their equity is tied up with their home. In recent years, equity release schemes have emerged and older people find themselves in situations where they make decisions about releasing their capital from the property or possibly selling it. These are difficult decisions because a home is more than a building where personal capital is tied up, it is composed of memories and represents a lifetime of achievement (Golant, 1998; Heywood *et al.*, 2002). Older people may feel that they have no other choice than to seek ways of releasing the money from their property, as they are unable to generate money from other sources. A member of the Expert Panel stated that:

> We have a lot of people in that situation *[unable to finance repairs to their house]* ... They then have to go back and release some of the funds from their property *[through equity release schemes]*.

The members of the Expert Panel argued that the root of the problem rested with the means-testing approach to determine whether an individual is or is not eligible for benefits. They suggested that a different, perhaps more graduated, approach to access benefits – rather than the sharp cut-off approach – would reduce the current inequity and that this would encourage younger people to continue to make financial arrangements for their later life.

Money and resources for a comfortable later life

While considerable attention has been given to the plight of older people who live on low incomes, Age Concern (2002a) highlighted in its policy position paper on income that average pensioner incomes had increased during the last 20 years, with those on high incomes tending to gain more. In 2001, 40 per cent of pensioners had incomes high enough to make them liable for income tax and 2 per cent were liable for the higher rate of tax (United Kingdom Parliament, House of Commons, 2001). These statistics indicate that there are older people in the UK who enter their later years with disposable income.

The older people who considered themselves to be 'financially well-off' or 'having a decent income' who took part in this study described how their financial circumstances affected their lives. They were no longer bound by the constraints of work commitments and they had buying power to realise personal objectives and aspirations. Some of the items that they spent their money on were:

- personal items such as clothing and mobile phones
- leisure and learning activities
- personal interests
- travel
- maintaining their home
- renewing household items
- services (such as domestic help) and equipment
- private health care
- gifts for family and friends
- intergenerational transfers of money (such as paying for their children's mortgages and grandchildren's education).

They argued that having money enabled them to continue to enjoy their life as they did prior to retirement and to participate fully in whatever was occurring in society. Many spoke of the way that they were able to give money to younger members of their family and how this elicited feelings of comfort and satisfaction. Their financial resources provided a sense of security and gave them a 'feeling of back-up' to cope with whatever changes they confronted in their later years.

According to George (1993), the value of income rests with its potential to be 'an empowering resource that fosters a sense of control' or 'an illusion of control' over one's circumstances (George, 1993, pp. 19–20). With money and health, an older person can make independent decisions about their lifestyle, maintain social contact and determine the extent to which they engage with the rest of society. This was epitomised in the following extract from the discussion between members of the Expert Panel:

> Finance is the key really. Well not only to retirement: it is at all levels. Those that have money are able to participate *[in]* its power really. So that you can choose how you want to live, if you haven't got money or are restricted in money you are very limited and you've got to have the sort of environment where people determine how *[you live]* ... You've no choice, have you?

Danigelis and McIntosh (2001) argued, however, that studies concerning financial satisfaction over-emphasised the importance of income. They drew on the earlier work of Arber and Ginn (1991) who placed monetary resources in the general category of material resources. Other material resources that older people possess include financial assets (for example, investments and pension plans), housing and car ownership. Of equal importance to material resources, but not directly monetary resources, they suggest that supportive and health-care resources (caring resources), and physical well-being and optimal functional abilities (health resources) form an interlocking 'Resource Triangle', in which different types of resources complement each other (Arber and Ginn 1991, p. 68).

Through the development of this model, non-monetary resources can be perceived as functional equivalents to monetary resources. An example of this would be where family members provide informal care or assistance with house maintenance where no financial transaction takes place. In this sense, Danigelis and McIntosh (2001) suggest that non-monetary resources might substitute for monetary resources in the minds of people when they consider their financial situation. With respect to the question 'Does money matter?' it may be argued that money is indeed important to the health and well-being of older people. However, this is only one of the resources that older people use in their daily lives and this ought to be taken into consideration in any appraisal of the importance of money in later life.

Financial resources: a mediator of disability, ill health and frailty

Levels of disability, ill health and functional dependence on others to meet personal needs as a consequence of frailty rise with increasing age. Around four million adults aged 65 and over (approximately a quarter of this group of people) report long-standing sickness or disability (Jarvis and Tinker, 1999; Palmer *et al.*, 2002). The direct and indirect costs associated with this for the individual and their family/carers are well reported. For example, Argyle's study of poverty, disability and older carers highlights the material costs of meeting living and caring expenses that include the payment of substitute care, purchase of domestic help, aids and adaptations to the home, special furniture, and specialised food and equipment (Argyle, 2001). Spending money on these items takes up much of the household income and erodes the older person's financial assets. In response to this, Argyle found that many people exercised financial caution when making decisions about what to spend their money on. Similar findings were derived from Whetstone's (2002) study, which documented the way in which low income compounds the effect that ill health and disability have on the older person's quality of life.

Local authorities are required to provide aids, adaptations and services to disabled people to enable them to live independent lives. Therefore, it could be argued that the direct costs of disability and chronic ill health will not be borne by the older person and their carers. There is evidence, however, that the processes of assessment of need (to determine eligibility for aids, equipment and adaptations to the home) are not responsive to the needs of older people and their carers. For example, a review of complaints by the Commission for Local Administration in England (1993) identified that there were unacceptable waiting times for the very items older people require to enable them to live in their own home. One consequence of this situation is that older people, if they have the money to do so, finance these items themselves (Age Concern, 1996). Those living in low-income households are unlikely to have sufficient money to pay for necessary equipment and assistance. In these situations, the practical demands that are made on the informal carer increase (Argyle, 2001). As one in four carers of older people is over retirement age themselves, this increases the physical, social and emotional burden of caring, which has an impact on the carer's health (Howard, 2001).

Older people who are living on modest incomes experience difficulties and worries about meeting the cost of care and assistance because they are required to make a contribution to their package of care. While this financial commitment may be problematic, other difficulties arise when the package of care exceeds the funding ceiling that is set by the local authority. In this situation, the older person can pay the full cost of additional care, which may outstrip their income, investments and assets. When they cannot meet the cost of the additional care, they face the decision to move to a care home.

These issues surface in the debate about payment for long-term care that has been a highly contentious topic in recent years. During the early 1990s, there were numerous reports in the press that the older generation was being subjected to asset stripping. Older people experienced great concern, not only about the move to care and what life would be like in a care home, but whether long-term care would be available to them if they were unable to pay for it. This culminated in the setting up of the Royal Commission on Long Term Care (United Kingdom Parliament, 1999), which set the background for changes to the regulations for the payment of long-term care. Concessions have been made in that health care is now differentiated from social care, but there remain many discussions about means testing and the payment of long-term care.

A central theme arising from the Expert Panel discussion and the key informant interviews was the importance of having money to purchase what was required to enable older people to maintain their independence. They argued that this was important because the prospect of becoming dependent on others for basic needs was greatly feared, as it threatened self-respect and eroded dignity. Personal stories were shared during these discussions to illustrate how the use of money promoted independence and enhanced the quality of life of those living with disabilities. One female key informant discussed how she had used her money to purchase an electronic scooter, which had been very costly. She had been housebound for some time and she indicated that being able to get out and about was liberating. She was able to meet with friends and she no longer felt lonely and depressed. She was able to do her shopping and messages. Throughout the discussion, she reflected on the positive impact that the scooter had made on her life, enabling her to experience a degree of satisfaction in life despite her physical limitations.

This evidence illustrates the interrelationships between the different types of resources – as identified in the Resource Triangle (Arber and Ginn, 1991) – that older people draw on in their day-to-day lives. Monetary resources can be used to compensate for lost functional abilities and to buy additional caring resources (see Clark *et al.*, 1998 for discussion of the importance of being able to pay for 'that little bit of help'). The value of monetary resources does not rest merely with the notion of purchasing power. Having access to this resource increases an older person's control over what is provided and when it is provided. Therefore, autonomy is enhanced. Those with limited monetary resources and diminished health resources are particularly vulnerable, as they are unable to compensate for lost functional abilities and place greater reliance on their care resources.

Giving control back to older people dependent on care: direct payments and brokerage schemes

The previous discussion highlighted the importance of independence to older people, which is associated with being able to make choices and to act on them (Collopy, 1988). Older people living with ill health and disability may lack the ability or freedom to carry out their decisions while retaining the capacity to make decisions. If they were able to make decisions about their life, they would exercise choice over how to live, from whom to get assistance and what their assistants would be required to do. In acknowledgement of this, direct payment and brokerage schemes have been developed to create a way of increasing service users' involvement in decisions about their life (United Kingdom Parliament, 1997; Hasler *et al.*, 1999).

Direct payments allow service users to be given direct funding to enable them to purchase help and support, as they need it, rather than having care packages imposed on them. As such, direct payment provides a means by which service users can be empowered in making decisions and having more control over the help they receive. The involvement of service users becomes central to the way that services are delivered, rather than minimal and marginal. For older people from ethnic groups, who may have needs and preferences not addressed by mainstream services, this could mean that services that are more acceptable to them are put in place.

Clark and Spafford (2001) have evaluated the direct payment scheme. They found that, while the scheme generally provided a high level of service, there were some barriers and problems, including the following.

- People did not take up the scheme because they had limited social networks and could not find people to do the caring. Some also found it a daunting prospect.
- Care managers found it difficult to take ownership of the scheme and did not have a support scheme.
- Minority ethnic groups had a low take-up.
- There were tensions between empowerment and protection – while the Social Services Department (SSD) wanted to promote choice and control for older people, it also wanted to ensure that they were not exploited or put at risk.

- The pilot benefited from proactive support from the SSD involved and from a proactive policy of offering the scheme to service users.

Clark and Spafford (2001) concluded that the pilot offered much to service users and potentially enhanced their choice and control over services. For some older people, the responsibilities of direct payment may be onerous and unwelcome, particularly in respect of accounting and employment responsibilities. This may be particularly the case if people are frail, have sight or hearing problems, are from ethnic groups, or might otherwise feel restricted in the degree to which they can engage with the processes of direct payment.

The brokerage scheme provided by Age Concern, Newcastle-upon-Tyne offers support and advice for people wanting to use direct payments to employ carers. The workers in the scheme offer support, for example, in drafting advertisements and job descriptions, managing the interview process and providing a 24-hour on-call service to address issues as they arise (e.g. gaps in care resulting from carers' sickness). The brokerage support can range from simply offering advice to carrying out the entire process on behalf of the service user. Hence, the responsibilities associated with managing direct payments are reduced for the older person and they can have as much involvement in decisions about their care as they desire. The rights of carers are upheld in this scheme because Age Concern takes on the employment of carers and assumes employer liability, as well as ensuring that the conditions of service are the same as other Age Concern employees.

These schemes provide mechanisms to involve older people in the decisions that affect their lives and to have choices. Although these are real benefits, there are risks, responsibilities and demands that older people must understand prior to making the transition to direct payment. Otherwise they may find that they have increased their vulnerability to their circumstances.

Contribution to society

Though older people who have entered retirement are generally regarded as not being able or being unable to make an economic contribution to society, the participants in the study challenged this. They argued that some older people continue to participate in the workforce while others make a non-monetary contribution to society. For example, many older people provide childcare for grandchildren, domestic work, voluntary work, informal care and learning activities, while also helping friends and neighbours. In addition, many older people participate in government committees set up specifically to involve them in priority-setting decisions for public spending.

A similar range of activities was identified by Barnes *et al.* (2002) when they explored the experiences and expectations of 48 people in their 50s and 60s. They also identified factors that influenced older people's participation outside of the labour market.

- Few interests were associated with heavy family care commitments, restricted mobility, recent bereavement and limited social networks.

- Many diverse interests were associated with the following factors – few family care commitments, good social networks, financial security, gradual withdrawal from work, strategies to plan for retirement and long-standing non-labour market interests and involvement.

The discussions with older people focused particularly on the contribution of older people as grandparents, volunteers, unpaid work in committees and informal care. The following discussions therefore focus on these topics.

Harper (2000) highlighted the way in which increasing longevity has had an impact on ties across the generations. Children are now more likely to have surviving grandparents and grandparents who are more likely to occupy this position for a longer proportion of their lives. An increasing number of older people provide childcare for their grandchildren, to enable their own children to work. In these situations, there may or may not be monetary exchanges and the activity serves to increase the interdependence between older and younger members of the family (Smith *et al.*, 2001). There is evidence that grandchildren benefit emotionally and cognitively from having a close relationship with a grandparent (Adkins,1999) and this may contribute to the older person's sense of well-being. Excessive demands to provide childcare, however, can have negative consequences, such as decreased social networking and increases in stress for the grandparent (Davidhizar *et al.*, 2000).

It is estimated that 50 per cent of the adult population of the UK volunteer at least once a year (Lynn and Davis Smith, 1991) and a significant proportion are older people. It has been found that the motivation behind volunteering is not just altruism, it may result from personal interest or merely response to direct requests. Volunteering also involves social benefits, wider social networks, physical and mental fitness, meaningful activity, a sense of purpose and new skills and experience (Dean and Morton, 1995; Krause and Shaw, 2000; Wardell *et al.*, 2000; Reed *et al.*, 2002). Volunteering, therefore, serves multiple purposes that meet the needs of those using and providing services. In recent years, policy makers have had high expectations of volunteers and voluntary organisations (Volunteering Unit, 1995) to increase their range of activity and contribution to service provision. Nonetheless, there are policy and contracting practices that present organisational barriers to the extended involvement of older volunteers. As the policy and regulatory framework for the voluntary sector is developing, careful consideration needs to be given to support and value the contribution of older volunteers to maintain their commitment to this type of activity.

Another form of volunteering has developed in recent years – that is, participating in committees to give the views of older people. There has been considerable emphasis on the involvement of older people in priority setting and service planning groups in recent government policy. From the perspective of the volunteers, this type of involvement is important, although it can equate to unpaid work. It is generally accepted that expenses will be met, but there are real hidden costs to participation, such as purchasing suitable clothing. If this type of activity is to be maintained and encouraged, it needs to be fully funded as a valuable and recognised activity.

The contribution of older people to the provision of unpaid care is significant. Older people are more likely to be spouse carers in contrast to younger carers and they are likely to spend long periods of time caring (Howard, 2001). For these reasons, the physical and emotional burden of care is considerable. The financial cost of care poses additional burdens, as there are extra care-related costs to meet, such as heating, clothing and laundry. In situations where alternative personal care is required, the older person may have to make a contribution to the package of care or to pay for this out of their savings. In situations where the older carer perceives that their financial situation has deteriorated, this has been attributed to the charges for services that they have faced (Holzausen and Pearlman, 2000).

This discussion has been an attempt to give illustrations of the ways in which older people make an important contribution to society. Often, the contribution is unrecognised, unpaid and unrewarded. This poses a major challenge: to rethink the way that making a contribution to society is conceptualised, to include both monetary and non-monetary contributions as valued resources.

4 Discussion

The themes and the literature that have been discussed represent the issues that are significant to the participants in this study. There is an extensive and diverse literature about these issues. However, much of what has been researched and written reflects the concerns of campaigners, academics, researchers and policy makers. For this reason, those who study older people and those who work on their behalf largely overshadow the voice of the older person in the literature. Consequently, there is a need to develop a body of knowledge that is grounded in the everyday experiences of older people and reflects their concerns and priorities.

Does money matter to older people?

Following examination of the question 'Does money matter to older people?', it has become apparent that it would be more appropriate to ask the questions 'how does money matter to older people?' and 'what difference does money make to the lives of older people?'. The overriding conclusion that can be drawn from the conversations that we have had with older people is that money is valued, not as an end in itself, but as a means to an end. The value of money rests in what it enables you to do and in the sense of financial security that it gives.

Having money – issues and concerns

An enjoyable and satisfying later life is one where there are possibilities to pursue goals and aspirations, and to have enough money to be able to meet the costs of living in modern society. These costs include more than being able to pay for the essentials of food, heating and clothing. The cost of living refers to having the money to access the range of resources that fellow citizens accept as essential commodities and the activities that others enjoy. Without the monetary resources to do this, older people experience exclusion from a society that is dominated by notions of consumerism. This highlights the importance of policy that encourages younger people to make financial decisions about planning for their later life and developing the necessary skills to effectively manage their monetary resources.

The concept of social inclusion also implies that you are able to make a contribution and that that contribution is valued. We have presented evidence that older people do make a significant contribution in many ways to society. However, their contribution is not always recognised. This is fertile ground for further investigation and there is a need to develop knowledge of means to facilitate older people to contribute to society in ways that they value.

An increasing proportion of those entering retirement have private and occupational pensions, financial assets and savings. These people have the potential to take advantage of the increasing range of leisure and educational opportunities that are available. Some, however, do not do this because they have concerns that the value of their income and financial assets will deteriorate as a consequence of poor indexing and of the possible need to pay for care if their health declines. As a consequence, they make financial decisions to maintain rather than use their financial resources, so as to ensure that they will have enough money for the remainder of their life.

While considerable attention has been given to understanding the needs and problems of those living on low incomes, little research has been carried out to understand the issues and concerns of those who have a modest if not a good income. This points to gaps in existing knowledge about how older people experience social inclusion and what helps or inhibits this from occurring. There is also a need for the development of support and independent advisory services to enable older people to make the best decisions about use of their money and to plan for the future. The development of policies for safeguarding older people's assets and their incomes needs further investigation from the perspective of older people because they are living at a time in their life when they are unable to generate additional income.

Involving those on low incomes in decisions about income

There has been extensive research and campaigning about the plight of older people who are living on low incomes. There is no doubt that the lives of older people living in these circumstances are harsh and impoverished. This is a grinding and never-ending experience. Acknowledgement of these circumstances has focused attention on improving the income of older people to enhance the quality of their lives. 'How much is enough money?' is a well-rehearsed political debate that will continue into the future. The older people that we spoke to were very articulate about this subject. They referred to the following ways of thinking about reaching conclusions about this.

1 What do older people need (as defined by objective criteria and by external assessors)?

2 What do older people want (as defined by subjective criteria and by older people themselves)?

3 How can we reach a compromise between 1 and 2?

Perhaps older people and the organisations that campaign on their behalf should be involved in defining what older people need and in developing ways in which to include them in the decision-making processes about what money they receive and how they access it. The introductions of the new tax credits and the transition to new ways of paying benefits through Automated Credit Transfer are recent initiatives that illustrate lack of consultation with the very groups that will be affected by these changes.

The literature that we reviewed highlighted the general dislike that older people have of the means-testing processes used to determine eligibility for welfare benefits and the problems associated with benefit take-up. These issues are well recognised and there are many campaigns to promote change to the way that benefits are accessed. Promoting change in ways that are appropriate and most acceptable to older people may reduce the problems of benefit take-up. This can be achieved only if it is known what benefits older people need and what they consider to be the most appropriate ways for them to receive the benefit. The development of this knowledge base needs to reflect the diverse circumstances of older people. For example, there are many older people from black and minority ethnic groups where English is their second language and they rely on the support of community and voluntary groups to assist them in the process of applying for benefits. Existing processes for claiming benefits require specialist knowledge and well-developed literacy skills to complete the relevant forms. Therefore, there is a requirement for greater knowledge of literacy levels among older people and the development of specialist services to support older people through the process of benefit application.

One response to the problems associated with benefit take-up has been the suggestion of giving universal benefits and universal concessions to older people. The key advantage to this is the minimisation of the stigma attached to the process of claiming benefits. However, this may not be the most effective, nor the best use of public money. In recognition of the finite budget that is available for public expenditure, it would be worthwhile developing a greater understanding of what older people value, what they will use and what they want. For example, the winter fuel payment is made to older people as one way of addressing the problem of fuel poverty in later life. However, there is still little understanding of older people's attitudes to central heating and heating their homes, nor do we fully understand why people have problems with paying their bills. While having money gives choice and a sense of control over one's circumstances, this has to be balanced with the social inclusion that universal concessions and benefits bring.

Paying for health and personal care services, aids, equipment and household adaptations

People are living longer and with advancing age there is an increased probability of need for services, aids and equipment to support independent living, or for long-term care. Those taking part in this study were greatly concerned with the issue of who pays for this. They expressed the opinion that the better-off older people have the financial resources to meet the costs of these services. In this way, they are able to identify what help they require and to control when and how help is provided. Those on low incomes, however, are reliant on the services and resources that are provided by health and social services. This situation contributes to service users feeling a lack of control over their circumstances and experiencing a degree of vulnerability: they feel that they are at the mercy of what is and what is not provided by the state.

To address the problem of diminished control, initiatives (such as direct payment and brokerage schemes) have been developed to promote the independence and autonomy of older people who are in receipt of services. These schemes do increase the involvement of service users in decisions about their care and how that care is provided, but this level of involvement incurs a range of responsibilities. The brokerage schemes strive to achieve a balance between facilitating involvement and enabling the older person to make decisions about the type of responsibilities that they are willing and able to fulfil. Evaluation of these schemes will highlight how older people view them and how they can be developed.

The way in which health and social care policy has developed in recent years has led to a situation where service users are increasingly being required to pay directly for personal social services or to be means tested to determine eligibility. The literature provides evidence to show that older people use much of their disposable income on purchasing services and resources, sometimes to the detriment of purchasing other essential items such as food and heating. The strategies that older people use to eke out their monetary resources, such as restricting levels and types of support, have been under-investigated. These need to be understood in order to prioritise service provision in the interests of older people.

The system for charging for personal care changed in October 2002. This introduced the principle that those with an income that exceeds the value of income support +30 per cent would now be eligible to make a contribution to the payment for their care. In some areas of the country, this resulted in large numbers of older people moving to the category of non-contributors and receiving free personal care services. This has had a major impact on the budgets of social services departments and it remains to be seen what influence these changes will have on the range and quantity of services provided by social services departments. The introduction of the new system of charging for care may result in increasing inequality throughout the country, as more people in affluent areas become eligible to make a personal contribution. There is also a concern that the new funding arrangements will lead to a focus on those requiring short-term care, while those with lesser and more sustained needs will be squeezed out of the priorities for service provision. If this situation arises, those who are living on low incomes may find that they will be expected to pay for a new range of necessary help and resources, or to live without them.

Paying for health and personal care services, aids, equipment and household adaptations has been a subject that has been given much consideration in the literature and in public debate. The issues that have been discussed here merely flag up some of the topics and the concerns of those that we were able to talk to during this study. The discussion, therefore, has not attempted to ignore other issues, such as the payment of long-term care or the subject of housing, which are equally important to the lives of older people. The issues that have been presented here focus on those that have been given minimal attention elsewhere in the literature.

Conclusion

The research team was charged with a mission to develop a 'think-piece' report, to provoke debate about the role of money in later life and to identify topics for future research. Throughout the development of this report, we were able to consult older people and those who are active in campaigning for them about the issues that were of greatest concern to them and this guided the processes of selecting and reviewing the literature. The review covered an extensive and diverse range of literature. This has been reported on in a way that presents the views of those who took part in the study alongside the views of those writing reports and articles concerning the question of whether money matters to older people in later life.

The overriding conclusion that was reached following review of the literature was that money is valued, not as an end, but as a means to an end. The value of money rests in what it enables you to do and in the sense of control over personal circumstances that it gives.

This study found that older people have major concerns about their income. They have entered a period of their life where there is little opportunity to increase their income. Indeed, some face the prospect of the real value of their income decreasing in the future as a result of poor indexation. In addition, the possibility of increased expenditure on paying for care, aids, equipment and adaptations to the home results in those affected experiencing financial insecurity in later life.

Older people are disproportionately represented in the lower income bracket. Considerable evidence has been presented in this report of the harsh conditions and the problems of living in these circumstances. These issues are well recognised in the literature and there are campaigns that are aimed at reducing pensioner poverty that, no doubt, will continue in the future. There is little written, however, from the perspective of older people about their priorities for change. More work needs to be done to capture these views and to develop ways to involve older people in decision making.

Bibliography

References (literature cited in the text of the report)

Adkins, V.K. (1999) 'Grandparents as a national asset: a brief note', *Activities, Adaptation and Aging*, Vol. 24, No. 1, pp. 13–8

Age Concern (1996) *Stuck on the Waiting List: Older People and Equipment for Independent Living. Age Concern National Campaign.* London: Age Concern

Age Concern (2001a) *The Pension Credit – Consultation Paper (DSS). Age Concern Comments.* Policy Paper, Ref. No. 1001. London: Age Concern

Age Concern (2001b) *Age Concern's Response to the Inland Revenue's Consultation Paper New Tax Credits.* Policy Paper, Ref. No. 2301. London: Age Concern

Age Concern (2002a) *Income. Policy Position Paper.* London: Age Concern

Age Concern (2002b) *Modest but Adequate. A Reasonable Living Standard for Households Aged 65–74. A Summary.* Policy Paper, Ref. No. 2304. London: Age Concern

Arber, S. and Ginn, J. (1991) *Gender and Later Life: A Sociological Analysis of Resources and Constraints.* London: Sage

Argyle, E. (2001) 'Poverty, disability and the role of older carers', *Disability and Society*, Vol. 16, No. 4, pp. 585–95

Atchley, R.C. (1997) 'Retirement income security: past, present, and future', *Generations*, Vol. 21, No. 2, pp. 9–12

Bardasi, E. and Jenkins, S.P. (2002) *Income in Later Life: Work History Matters.* Bristol: Policy Press in conjunction with Joseph Rowntree Foundation

Barnes, H., Parry, J. and Lakey, J. (2002) *Forging a New Future: The Experiences and Expectations of People Leaving Paid Work over 50.* Bristol: Policy Press

Bartlett, A. (2001) *Financial Planning: An Examination of Women's Special Needs.* PRA Research Seminar, September, London. PRA Occasional Paper. Guildford: Pre-retirement Association (PRA)

Beresford, P., Green, D., Lister, R. and Woodard, K. (1999) *Poverty First Hand – Poor People Speak for Themselves.* London: White Lion Street in conjunction with the Child Poverty Action Group.

Bradshaw, J. (2000) 'Prospects for poverty in Britain in the first twenty-five years of the next century', *Sociology – the Journal of the British Sociological Association*, Vol. 34, No. 1, pp. 53–70

Bramley, G., Lancaster, S. and Gordon, D. (2000) 'Benefit take-up and the geography of poverty in Scotland', *Regional Studies*, Vol. 34, No. 6, pp. 507–19

Bryant, L.L., Corbett, K.K. and Kutner, J.S. (2001) 'In their own words: a model of healthy aging', *Social Science and Medicine*, Vol. 53, No. 7, pp. 927–41

Chang, D., Spicer, N., Irving, A., Sparham, I. and Neeve, L. (2001) *Modernising Service Delivery: The Better Government for Older People Prototypes.* Department for Work and Pensions Research Report No. 136. London: Department for Work and Pensions

Clark, H. and Spafford, J. (2001) *Piloting Choice and Control for Older People: An Evaluation.* Bristol: Policy Press

Clark, H., Dyer, S. and Horwood, J. (1998) *That Bit of Help: The High Value of Low Level Preventative Sevices for Older People.* York: Joseph Rowntree Foundation

Collopy, B.J. (1988) 'Autonomy in long-term care: some crucial distinctions', *The Gerontologist*, Vol. 28, June (supplement), pp. 10–17

Commission for Local Administration in England (Local Government Ombudsman) (1993) *Report on Investigation No. 9\A\1173 into a Complaint against the London Borough of Redbridge 9\12\93.* London: Commission for Local Administration in England (Local Government Ombudsman)

Corden, A. (1995) *New Perspectives on Take-up: A Literature Review.* SPRU (Social Policy Research Unit). London: HMSO

Costigan, P., Finch, H., Jackson, B., Legard, R. and Ritchie, J. (1999) *Overcoming Barriers: Older People and Income Support.* Department for Work and Pensions Research Report No. 100. London: Department for Work and Pensions

Cutler, N.E. (1997) 'The false alarms and blaring sirens of financial literacy: middle-agers' knowledge of retirement income, health finance, and long-term care', *Generations*, Vol. 21, No. 2, pp. 34–40

Danigelis, N.L. and McIntosh, B.R. (2001) 'Gender's effect on the relationships linking older Americans' resources and financial satisfaction', *Research on Aging*, Vol. 23, No. 4, pp. 410–28

Davidhizar, R., Bechtel, G.A. and Woodring, B.C. (2000) 'The changing role of grandparenthood', *Journal of Gerontological Nursing*, Vol. 26, No. 1, pp. 24–9

Dean, J. and Morton, M. (1995) *A Chance to Help: Survey of Later Life Volunteers in Scotland.* Stirling: Volunteer Development Scotland

Department for Education and Employment (1999) *Improving Literacy and Numeracy: A Fresh Start.* The report of the Working Group on Post-school Basic Skills chaired by Sir Claus Moser. London: Department for Education and Employment

Department of Works and Pensions (2001) *The Pensioners' Income Series 1999/00.* London: Department of Works and Pensions, Analytical Services Division

Disney, R., Grundy, E. and Johnson, P. (eds) (1978) *The Dynamics of Retirement. Analyses of the Retirement Surveys.* Department for Work and Pensions Research Report No. 72. London: Department for Work and Pensions

Disney, R., Johnson, P. and Stears, G. (1998) 'Asset wealth and asset decumulation among households in the retirement survey', *Fiscal Studies,* Vol. 19, No. 2, pp. 153–74

Evandrou, M. and Falkingham, J. (1993) 'Social security and the life course, developing sensitive policy alternatives', in S. Arber and M. Evandrou (eds) *Ageing, Independence and the Life Course.* London: Jessica Kingsley

Evans, M. and Falkingham, J. (1997) *Minimum Pensions and Safety Nets in Old Age: A Comparative Analysis.* Suntory and Toyota International Centre for Economics and Related Disciplines (STICERD). London: London School of Economics and Political Science

Ferraro, K.F. and Su, Y. (1999) 'Financial strain, social relations, and psychological distress among older people: a cross-cultural analysis', *Journals of Gerontology, Series B – Psychological Sciences and Social Sciences,* Vol. 54B, No. 1, pp. S3–S15

Financial Services Authority (1998) *Promoting Public Understanding of Financial Services: A Strategy for Consumer Education.* London: Financial Services Authority

Flately, J. (1999) *Helping Pensioners: Contextual Survey of the Income Support Pilots.* Department for Work and Pensions In-house Report No. 60. London: Department for Work and Pensions

George, L.K. (1992) 'Economic status and subjective well being: a review of the literature and an agenda for future research', in N.A. Cutler, D.W. Gregg and M.P. Lawton (eds) *Ageing, Money and Life Satisfaction.* New York: Springer

George, L.K. (1993) *Financial Security in Later Life: The Subjective Side.* Philadelphia, PA: Boettner Institute of Financial Gerontology

Gnich, W. and Gilhooly, M. (1997) 'Financial planning and financial well-being in later life', poster presentation, British Society of Gerontology Annual Conference, September

Gnich, W. and Gilhooly, M. (2001) 'Planning for financial well-being in old age: an investigation of baby boomers and older adults in Scotland' (abstract), *The Gerontologist*, Vol. 41, No. 1, p. 143

Golant, S.M. (1998) 'Changing an older person's shelter and care setting: a model to explain personal and environmental outcomes', in R.J. Scheidt and P.G. Windley (eds) *Environment and Ageing Territory. A Focus on Housing*. Westport CT: Greenwood Press

Gordon, D., Adelman, L., Ashworth, K., Bradshaw, J., Levitas, R., Middleton, S., Pantazis, C., Patsios, D., Payne, S., Townsend, P. and Williams, J. (2000) *Poverty and Social Exclusion in Britain*. York: Joseph Rowntree Foundation

Harper, S. (2000) 'Locating grandparents', in A. Dickinson, H. Bartlett and S. Wade (eds) *Old Age in a New Age. Proceedings of the British Society of Gerontology Annual Conference, 8–10 September 2000, Keble College, Oxford*. Oxford: Oxford Brookes University

Hasler, F., Campbell, J. and Zarb, G. (1999) *Direct Routes to Independence: A Guide to Local Authority Implementation and Management of Direct Payments*. London: Policy Studies Institute

Hedges, A. (1998) *Pensions and Retirement Planning*. Department for Work and Pensions Research Report No. 83. London: Department for Work and Pensions

Heywood, F., Oldman, C. and Means, R. (2002) *Housing and Home in Later Life*. Buckingham: Open University Press

Holzausen, E. and Pearlman, V. (2000) *Caring on the Breadline: The Financial Implications of Caring*. London: Carers' National Association

Howard, M. (2001) *Paying the Price: Carers, Poverty and Social Exclusion*. Child Poverty Action Group in association with Carers UK. London: Russell Press

Howarth, C., Kenway, P. and Palmer, C. (2001) *Responsibility for All: A National Strategy for Social Inclusion*. London: New Policy Institute, Fabian Society

Humphrey, R. and Calder, J. (1990) *Resilience or Resignation? Retirement and Unmet Need in the West End of Newcastle*. Newcastle-Upon-Tyne: Search Project

Jarvis, C. and Tinker, A. (1999) 'Trends in old age morbidity and disability in Britain', *Ageing and Society*, Vol. 19, No. 5, pp. 603–27

Johnson, P., Stears, G. and Webb, S. (1998) 'The dynamics of incomes and occupational pensions after retirement', *Fiscal Studies*, Vol. 19, No. 2, pp. 197–215

Kempson, E. and Whyley, C. (2001) *Well Enough to Work? Payment of Pensions and Benefits: A Survey of Social Security Recipients Paid by Order Book or Girocheque*. Department for Work and Pensions Research Report No. 146. London: Department for Work and Pensions

Kempson, E., Collard, S. and Taylor, S. (2002) *Social Fund Use among Older People in Britain*. Department for Work and Pensions Research Report No. 172. London: Department for Work and Pensions

Krause, N. (1997) 'Anticipated support, received support, and economic stress among older adults', *Journals of Gerontology, Series B – Psychological Sciences and Social Sciences*, Vol. 52B, No. 6, pp. P284–93

Krause, N. and Shaw, B.A. (2000) 'Giving social support to others, socioeconomic status, and changes in self-esteem in late life', *Journals of Gerontology, Series B – Psychological Sciences and Social Sciences*, Vol. 55B, No. 6, pp. S323–33

Lord, N. (2001) *Summing Up: Bridging the Financial Literacy Divide*. A CAB Evidence Report. London: National Association of Citizens Advice Bureaux

Lynn, P. and Davis Smith, J. (1991) *The 1991 National Survey of Voluntary Activity in the UK*. Berkhamsted: The Volunteer Centre UK

Marmot, M. and Wilkinson, R.G. (2001) 'Psychosocial and material pathways in the relation between income and health: a response to Lynch *et al.*', *British Medical Journal*, Vol. 322, No. 7296, pp. 1233–6

Mein, G., Higgs, P., Ferrie, J. and Stansfeld, S.A. (1998) 'Paradigms of retirement: the importance of health and ageing in the Whitehall II study', *Social Science and Medicine*, Vol. 47, No. 4, pp. 535–45

Mein, G., Martikainen, P., Stansfeld, S.A., Brunner, E.J., Fuhrer, R. and Marmot, M.G. (2000) 'Predictors of early retirement in British civil servants', *Age and Ageing*, Vol. 29, No. 6, pp. 529–36

Monroe, F. and Marks, S. (2002) *The Fuel Picture. CAB Clients' Experiences of Dealing with Fuel Suppliers*. CAB Evidence Report. London: National Association of Citizens Advice Bureaux

NHS CRD (Centre for Reviews and Dissemination) (2001) *Undertaking Systematic Reviews of Research on Effectiveness. CRD's Guidance for those Carrying out or Commissioning Reviews*. CRD Report No. 4, 2nd edn. York: CRD. http://www.york.ac.uk/inst/crd/report4.htm (accessed 10 February 2003)

NIACE (2001) *Adult Financial Literacy Advisory Group (AdFLAG) Report. A Response from NIACE on the AdFLAG Report to the Secretary of State for Education and Employment*. Leicester: NIACE

NIACE (2002) *Financial Literacy and Older People – Moving on*. NIACE Briefing Sheet No. 31. Leicester: NIACE

Ozawa, M.N. and Lum, Y. (1997) 'Economic satisfaction among American retirees', *Journal of Gerontological Social Work*, Vol. 27, No. 4, pp. 21–40

Ozawa, M.N. and Lum, Y. (1998) 'Marital status and change in income status ten years after retirement', *Social Work Research*, Vol. 22, No. 2, pp. 116–28

Palmer, G., Rahman, M. and Kenway, P. (2002) *Monitoring Poverty and Social Exclusion*. York: Joseph Rowntree Foundation

Parker, H. (ed.) (2000) *Low Cost but Acceptable Incomes for Older People: A Minimum Income Standard for Households Aged 65–74 Years in the UK*. Bristol: Policy Press

Parker, H. (ed.) (2002) *Modest but Adequate: A Reasonable Living Standard for Households Aged 65–74*. Study commissioned by Age Concern. York: Family Budget Unit, Social Policy Research Unit, University of York

Pre-retirement Association (2000) *Financial Education Project: A Report from the Pre-retirement Association*. Guildford: Pre-retirement Association

Prestoy, S.F. (1993) 'Quality of life as perceived and experienced through activity, relationships and sense of independence: an ethnography of seven urban older adults who attend a senior citizens' center', Doctor of Philosophy in the School of Education, Health, Nursing, and the Arts Profession, New York University, New York

Reed, J., Cook, G. and Stanley, D. (2002) *Help the Aged – Good Practice Report*. Centre for the Care of Older People. Newcastle-upon-Tyne: Northumbria University

Rooney, S. (2002) *Payment of Tax Credit and Benefits via Bank Accounts: A Review of Availability and Access in Washington*. Washington (UK): Washington Citizens Advice Bureau

Smith, C.J., Beltran, A., Butts, D.M. and Kingson, E.R. (2001) 'Grandparents raising grandchildren: emerging program and policy issues for the 21st century', *Journal of Gerontological Social Work*, Vol. 35, No. 1, pp. 33–45

United Kingdom Parliament (1997) *Statutory Instrument 1997 No. 734. The Community Care (Direct Payments) Regulations 1997*. London: HMSO

United Kingdom Parliament (1999) *With Respect to Old Age: Long Term Care – Rights and Responsibilities*. A Report by The Royal Commission on Long Term Care. Chairman: Professor Sir Stewart Sutherland. Cm. 4192-I. London: The Stationery Office

United Kingdom Parliament, House of Commons (2001) *Hansard*, Vol. 363 (House of Commons Debates). Written answers to questions. Pensioners (tax), 26 February, col. 518W

Villa, V.M., Wallace, S.P. and Markides, K. (1997) 'Economic diversity and an aging population: the impact of public policy and economic trends', *Generations*, Vol. 21, No. 3, pp. 13–18

Volunteering Unit (1995) *Make a Difference: An Outline Volunteering Strategy for the UK*. London: HMSO

Walker, J. and Davies, M. (2001) *Financial Literacy in Later Life. PRA Research Seminar, September 2001, London*. PRA Occasional Paper. Guildford: Pre-retirement Association

Walker, R., Heaver, C. and McKay, S. (2000) *Building up Pension Rights*. Department for Work and Pensions Research Report No. 114. London: Department for Work and Pensions

Walters, V. and Charles, N. (1997) '"I just cope from day to day": unpredictability and anxiety in the lives of women', *Social Science and Medicine*, Vol. 45, No. 11, pp. 1729–39

Wardell, F., Lishman, J. and Whalley, L.J. (2000) 'Who volunteers?', *British Journal of Social Work*, Vol. 30, pp. 227–48

Whetstone, M. (2002) *Hard Times. A Study of Pensioner Poverty*. CPA Report 31. London: Centre for Policy on Ageing (CPA)

Further reading (literature which provided contextual background to the project but which is not cited in the text of the report)

Age Concern (2002a) *Age Concern's Submission to the Work and Pension Committee Inquiry into the Future of Pensions*. Policy Paper, Ref. No. 2102. London: Age Concern

Age Concern (2002b) *Concerned about Ageing? The Needs of Older People: Key Issues and Evidence*. Policy Paper, Ref. No. 0202. London: Age Concern

Baldock, C.V. (1999) 'Seniors as volunteers: an international perspective on policy', *Ageing and Society*, Vol. 19, No. 5, pp. 581–602

Barton, A. (2002) *Unfair and Underfunded. CAB Evidence on What's Wrong with the Social Fund*. CAB Evidence Report. London: National Association for Citizens Advice Bureaux

Bennett, M., Smith, E., Victor, C.R. and Millard, P.H. (2000) 'The right person? The right place? The right time? A pilot study of the appropriateness of nursing home placements', *Archives of Gerontology and Geriatrics*, Vol. 31, No. 1, pp. 55–64

Blundell, R. and Johnson, P. (1998) 'Pensions and labor-market participation in the United Kingdom', *American Economic Review (AEA) Papers and Proceedings*, Vol. 88, pp. 168–72

Blundell, R. and Preston, I. (1995) 'Income, expenditure and the living standards of UK households', *Fiscal Studies*, Vol. 16, No. 3, pp. 40–54

Brandon, D., Maglajilic, R. and Given, D. (2000) 'Direct payments: the information deficit', *Working with Older People*, Vol. 4, No. 3, pp. 26–7

Brunell, M. (2001) 'Doing for others: it gives me something to do. An ethnographic study of older, urban women living alone in poverty', Columbia University Teachers' College, EdD

Carlton, S. and Soulsby, J. (1999) *Learning to Grow Older and Bolder. A Policy Discussion Paper on Learning in Later Life*. Leicester: NIACE

Carlton, S., Soulsby, J. and Whitelegg, D. (2002). *Old Money. Financial Understanding for Older Adult Learners*. Leicester: NIACE

Choi, N.G. (2000) 'Determinants of engagement in paid work following Social Security benefit receipt among older women', *Journal of Women and Aging*, Vol. 12, Nos 3/4, pp. 133–54

Clark, H. (2001) 'Direct Payments: the crucial role of support workers', *Working with Older People*, Vol. 5, No. 2, pp. 19–22

Corden, A. (1995) *Changing Perspectives on Benefit Take-up*. SPRU (Social Policy Research Unit), University of York. London, HMSO

Cutler, N.E. (1997) 'Introduction: financial dimensions of aging – and middle-aging', *Generations*, Vol. 21, No. 2, pp. 5–8

Daly, M. and Lewis, J. (2000) 'The concept of social care and the analysis of contemporary welfare states', *British Journal of Sociology*, Vol. 51, No. 2, pp. 281–98

Devlin, S.J. and Arye, L. (1997) 'The Social Security debate: a financial crisis or a new retirement paradigm?', *Generations*, Vol. 21, No. 2, pp. 27–33

Eldred, J. (2002) *Moving on with Confidence*. Leicester: NIACE

Fronstin, P. (1999) 'Retirement patterns and employee benefits: do benefits matter?', *The Gerontologist*, Vol. 39, No. 1, pp. 37–47

Gall, T.L., Evans, D.R. and Howard, J. (1997) 'The retirement adjustment process: changes in the well-being of male retirees across time', *Journals of Gerontology, Series B – Psychological Sciences and Social Sciences*, Vol. 52B, No. 3, pp. 110–17

Gilhooly, M. and Gnich, W. (2001) 'Ageing and financial well-being in Scotland: an investigation of the relationship between financial status, financial well-being, and health', *The Gerontologist*, Vol. 41, No. 1, p. 231

Gordon, B., Macdonald, S., Gilhooly, M., Hanlon, P. and Whyte, B. (2001) 'Psychosocial resources for good health and successful ageing', *The Gerontologist*, Vol. 41, No. 1, p. 136

Gow, J., Webster, N., Gilhooly, M., Hamilton, K., O'Neill, M., Edgerton, E. and Pike, F. (2001) 'Transport, aging and quality of life: findings from qualitative aspects of a comparative study', *The Gerontologist*, Vol. 41, No. 1, p. 231

Hales, J. and Stratford, N. (2000) *Employers' Pension Provision 1998*. Department for Work and Pensions Research Report No. 123. London: Department for Work and Pensions

Hancock, R., Katbamna, S., Martin, G., Clarke, H. and Stuchbury, R. (2002) *Attitudes to Inheritance: An Exploratory Study*. York: YPS for the Joseph Rowntree Foundation

Harding, T., Meredith, B. and Wistow, G. (eds) (1996) *Options for Long Term Care – Economic, Social, and Ethical Choices*. London: HMSO

Hayward, M.D., Friedman, S. and Chen, H. (1998) 'Career trajectories and older men's retirement', *Journals of Gerontology, Series B – Psychological Sciences and Social Sciences*, Vol. 53B, No. 2, pp. S91–103

Help the Aged (2002) *Tackling Pensioner Poverty Today*. Help the Aged Policy Statement, May 2002. London: Help The Aged

Hornstein, Z. (2001) *Outlawing Age Discriminatin: Foreign Lessons, UK Choices*. Bristol: Policy Press

Hutton, S., Williams, J. and Kennedy, S. (1997) *Women's Current Pension Arrangements: Information from the General Household Survey*. Department for Work and Pensions In-house Report No. 22. London: Department for Work and Pensions

Jansen, D.A. and Keller, M.L. (1998) 'Identifying the attentional demands perceived by elderly people', *Rehabilitation Nursing*, Vol. 23, No. 1, pp. 12–20, 56

Jerrome, D. and Wenger, G.C. (1999) 'Stability and change in late-life friendships', *Ageing and Society*, Vol. 19, pp. 661–76

Kawachi, I., Kennedy, B. and Wilkinson, R.G. (eds) (1999) *Income Inequality and Health: A Reader*. New York: New Press

Kelly, N.R. and Swisher, L. (1998) 'The transitional process of retirement for nurses', *Journal of Professional Nursing*, Vol. 14, No. 1, pp. 53–61

Kington, R.S. and Smith, J.P. (1997) 'Socioeconomic status and racial and ethnic differences in functional status associated with chronic diseases', *American Journal of Public Health*, Vol. 87, No. 5, pp. 805–10

Kubik, M.J. (1998) 'Is your financial house in order?', *Advanced Practice Nursing Quarterly*, Vol. 3, No. 4, pp. 14-22

Lobmayer, P. and Wilkinson, R. (2000) 'Income, inequality and mortality in 14 developed countries', *Sociology of Health and Illness*, Vol. 22, No. 4, pp. 401–14

Macdonald, S., Gordon, B., Gilhooly, M., Hanlon, P. and Whyte, B. (2001) 'Determinants of good health and successful ageing', *The Gerontologist*, Vol. 41, No. 1, p. 136

McGuinness, M. (1997) 'Recognising the financial abuse of older people', *Professional Nurse*, Vol. 12, No. 4, pp. 256–8

Manchester, J. (1997) 'Aging boomers and retirement: who is at risk?', *Generations*, Vol. 21, No. 2, pp. 19–22

Marks, S. (2002) *Door to Door: CAB Clients' Experience of Doorstep Selling*. London: National Association of Citizens Advice Bureaux

Mayhew, V. (2001) *Public Attitudes to Pensions and Planning for Retirement*. Department for Work and Pensions Research Report No. 130. London: Department for Work and Pensions

Mustard, C., Finlayson, M., Derksen, S. and Berthelot, J. (1999) 'What determines the need for nursing home admission in a universally insured population?', *Journal of Health Services and Research Policy*, Vol. 4, No. 4, pp. 197–203

Ozawa, M.N. (1999) 'The economic well-being of elderly people and children in a changing society', *Social Work*, Vol. 44, No. 1, pp. 9–19

Paulin, G.D. (2000) 'Expenditure patterns of older Americans, 1984–97', *Monthly Labor Review*, Vol. 123, No. 5, pp. 3–28

Pendry, E., Barrett, G. and Victor, C. (1999) 'Changes in household composition among the over sixties: a longitudinal analysis of the Health and Lifestyles Surveys', *Health and Social Care in the Community*, Vol. 7, No. 2, pp. 109–19

Rowlingson, K. (2000) *Fate, Hope and Insecurity: Future Orientation and Forward Planning*. York: Policy Studies Institute in association with the Joseph Rowntree Foundation

Rowlingson, K., Whyley, C. and Warren, T. (1999) *Wealth in Britain: A Lifecycle Perspective*. York: Policy Studies Institute in association with the Joseph Rowntree Foundation

Scharf, T., Phillipson, C., Smith, A.E. and Kingston, P. (2002) *Growing Older in Socially Deprived Areas: Social Exclusion in Later Life*. London: Help The Aged

Smith, G.C. and Sylvestre, G.M. (2001) 'Determinants of the travel behavior of the suburban elderly', *Growth and Change*, Vol. 32, No. 3, pp. 395–412

Suto, W.M.I., Holland, A.J., Clare, I.C.H. and Watson, P.C. (2000) 'Financial autonomy among adults with intellectual disability: the findings from a prevalence study', *Journal of Intellectual Disability Research*, Vol. 44, Nos 3–4, p. 1125

Tanner, S. (1998) 'The dynamics of male retirement behaviour', *Fiscal Studies*, Vol. 19, No. 2, pp. 175–96

Thomas, A. and Pettigrew, N. (1999) *Attitudes towards Method of Paying Benefits*. Department for Work and Pensions In-house Report No. 51. London: Department for Work and Pensions

Thomas, A., Pettigrew, N. and Tovey, P. (1999) *Increasing Compulsory Pension Benefits: Attitude of the General Public and the Self-employed.* Department for Work and Pensions In-house Report No. 48. London: Department for Work and Pensions

Toughill, E., Mason, D.J., Beck, T.L. and Christopher, M.A. (1993) 'Health, income, and postretirement employment of older adults', *Public Health Nursing*, Vol. 10, No. 2, pp. 100–7

Veit-Wilson, J. (2002) 'States of welfare: a response to Charles Atherton', *Social Policy and Administration*, Vol. 36, No. 3, pp. 312–17

Veit-Wilson, J. (2000) 'States of welfare: a conceptual challenge', *Social Policy and Administration*, Vol. 34, No. 1, pp. 1–25

Vernon, S., Ross, F. and Gould, M.A. (2000) 'Assessment of older people: politics and practice in primary care', *Journal of Advanced Nursing*, Vol. 31, No. 2, pp. 282–7

Walsh, K. and Bennett, G. (2000) 'Financial abuse of older people', *Journal of Adult Protection*, Vol. 2, No. 1, pp. 21–9

Warner, B. (1998) 'It's about time ... saving now for later', *ASHA* (Journal of the American Speech-Language-Hearing Association), Vol. 40, No. 2, pp. 36–42

Wieland, D., Lamb, V.L., Sutton, S.R., Boland, R., Clark, M., Friedman, S., Brummel-Smith, K. and Eleazer, G.P. (2000) 'Hospitalization in the Program of All-inclusive Care for the Elderly (PACE): rates, concomitants, and predictors', *Journal of the American Geriatrics Society*, Vol. 48, No. 11, pp. 1373–80

Zimmerman, L., Mitchell, B., Wister, A. and Gutman, G. (2000) 'Unanticipated consequences: a comparison of expected and actual retirement timing among older women', *Journal of Women and Aging*, Vol. 12, Nos 1/2, pp. 109–28

Appendix: Money matters literature search

See overleaf for appendix.

Table A1.1 Mapping of search terms across databases, Part 1

		Database and date searched						
Set no.	**Search term**	**PubMED (28.8.02)**	**AMED (28.8.02)**	**CINAHL, 1982–97 (28.8.02)**	**CINAHL, 1998–2002 (28.8.02)**	**Cochrane controlled trials, 2nd qtr 2002 (28.8.02)**	**Cochrane systematic reviews database (28.8.02)**	**Combined (28.8.02)**
1	Older people	27,751	301	205	1,312	96	60	1,974
2	Elderly people	266,239	228	131	531	137	48	1,075
3	Geriatric	265,370	308	257	1,233	410	66	2,274
4	Geriatrics	1,151	119	98	351	27	9	604
5	Retired	975	29	31	118	22	12	212
6	Retirement	1,309	51	101	519	17	12	700
7	Senior citizen	36	2	1	9	1	0	13
8	Senior citizens	104	17	13	52	3	0	85
9	Pensioner	8	0	0	4	0	0	4
10	Pensioners	30	3	1	9	0	2	15
11	1–10 (or)	276,909	925	766	3,824	636	143	6,294
12	Money	1,598	56	149	850	71	35	1,161
13	Income	9,633	161	308	1,758	235	70	2,532
14	Incomes	5,717	14	20	128	13	2	177
15	Expenditure	4,258	175	125	525	274	49	1,148
16	Spending	829	31	42	271	15	12	371
17	Financial	57,888	250	328	1798	131	281	2,788
18	Finances	66,132	24	18	106	7	5	160
19	Payment	1,801	51	86	656	25	23	841

(continued)

Table A1.1 Mapping of search terms across databases, Part 1 (continued)

		Database and date searched						
Set no.	**Search term**	**PubMED (28.8.02)**	**AMED (28.8.02)**	**CINAHL, 1982–97 (28.8.02)**	**CINAHL, 1998–2002 (28.8.02)**	**Cochrane controlled trials, 2nd qtr 2002 (28.8.02)**	**Cochrane systematic reviews database (28.8.02)**	**Combined (28.8.02)**
20	Payments	687	23	34	218	10	15	300
21	Benefits	19,291	1,032	798	4,706	1,860	856	9,252
22	Purchasing	752	38	53	220	13	14	338
23	12–22 (or)	81,931	1,733	1,810	10,345	2,567	143	17,534
24	11 and 23	16,474	70	76	320	33	86	585

Note: Limits imposed (where allowed by database) English language, date from 1997 and, in the case of PubMED, Human.

Table A1.2 Mapping of search terms across databases, Part 2

Set no.	Search term	Database and date searched SSCI (5.11.02)
1	Older people	2,895
2	Elderly people	2,577
3	Geriatric	5,313
4	Geriatrics	917
5	Retired	642
6	Retirement	3371
7	Senior citizen	68
8	Senior citizens	180
9	Pensioner	16
10	Pensioners	120
25	Financial literacy	5
26	Finance and advocacy	10
27	Financial strategies	12
28	Basic income	24
29	Minimal income	2
30	Basic needs	128
31	Income and autonomy	70
32	Financial autonomy	8
33	Financial gerontology	3
34	Financial well-being	9
35	Budget management	4
36	Personal budgets	1
37	Budget standards	2
38	Spending patterns	27
39	Social care and money or finances	390
40	Social exclusion and money or finances	394

Notes:	
Geriatric and 39	1
Geriatric and 40	0
Articles by:	
Bradshaw, J.	0
Femister, G.	0
Gilhooly, M.	14
Hill, M.	0
Townsend, P.	0
Veit-Wilson, J.	3
Younge, M.	0

(Continued)

Cited references:

Bradshaw, J.	181
After keyword searching for 'elderly'	12
Femister, G.	0
Gilhooly, M.	0
Hill, M.	0
Townsend, P.	0
Veit-Wilson, J.	0
Younge, M.	0